My
Health & Wellness
Organizer

An Easy Guide To Manage Your Healthcare—
and Your Medical Records

by
Puja A. J. Thomson

2022 Revised Edition

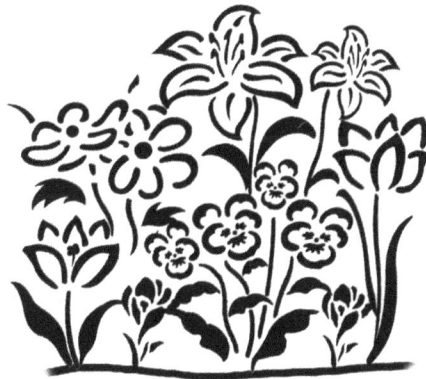

If found, please contact me and/or return to:

Name_____ Tel_____

Email: _____ Address:_____

1. Health   2. Self-help

Revised Edition 2022   ISBN 978-1-928663-14-0

Published by—ROOTS & WINGS, New Paltz, NY. Printed in the USA

Edited by—Johanna Bard

Design—Tory Ettlinger

Logo design—Helene Sarkis

Please note: This organizer is designed with the understanding that the author and publisher are not engaged in rendering individualized professional services. The suggestions, explorations and questions are intended for individual use and are not designed to be a substitute for professional consultation.

Other works by Puja A. J. Thomson:

Track Your Truth—Discover Your Authentic Self

My Hope & Focus Cancer Organizer (Second revised edition 2022)

After Shock: From Cancer Diagnosis to Healing (Second revised edition 2021)

Roots & Wings for Strength and Freedom—Guided Imagery And Meditations To Transform Your Life (CD and MP3)

Roots & Wings Workbook—Guided Imagery And Meditations To Transform Your Life
(Workbook & CD)

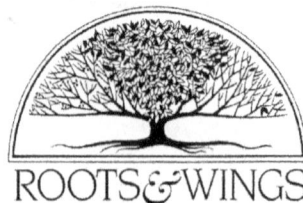

ROOTS&WINGS

To order any of the above titles or for general inquiries:

845-255-2278

ROOTS & WINGS PUBLISHING, P. O. Box 1081, New Paltz, NY 12561 Email: info@rootsnwings.com

www.rootsnwings.com/store

CONTENTS

Foreword

Patients often leave my office and lose the benefits of the treatment by having to deal with insurance companies, as well as trying to locate old records and keep track of the new ones that accumulate so rapidly.

In our technological medical world, when chronic disease or unexpected illness strikes, we are left disempowered and often feel helpless as to what we can do to support our healing process. Puja Thomson has gifted us with not only her deep wisdom, but just as importantly, a step by step practical guide to organize our journey to wellness.

In my own practice as an acupuncturist and herbalist, I see patients constantly grappling not only with their illnesses, but also with the chaos the illness brings with it. A chronic arthritic complaint, an auto-immune disease, or cancer, may bring them in for treatment. However patients often leave my office and lose the benefits of the treatment by having to deal with insurance companies, as well as trying to locate old records and keep track of the new ones that accumulate so rapidly. As we are working to create a clear and relaxed place to allow healing, these worries add more stress.

I am delighted that there is now an organizer which benefits not only those dealing personally with illness, but their families and friends as well. *My Health & Wellness Organizer* is indeed "an easy guide to manage your medical records." It provides a clear structure so that all your bills, forms, phone numbers, past health and current treatment information will be available immediately at your fingertips in a simple three-ring binder.

By using this powerful road map to organize your information and resources, you can create clarity out of chaos, and focus on healing.

Allow this book to support your health and simplify your life.

Jason Elias MA, LMT, LAc, DIPL. OM, *and author of* Feminine Healing, The A to Z Guide to Herbal Remedies *and* Chinese Medicine for Maximum Immunity

Acknowledgements

Many thanks go to Johanna Bard (*Your Hudson Valley Organizer*), Tory Ettlinger (*Ettlinger Design*), and Barbara Sarah (Founder of the Oncology Support Program of *The Health Alliance of the Hudson Valley*). This superb trio of creative women has been an unfailing source of support for me throughout the gestation and birth of **My Hope & Focus Cancer Organizer**. This laid the groundwork for **My Health & Wellness Organizer** which is appropriate for any health challenge. I am grateful for their continued guidance, skill and encouragement.

When invited to share his perspective as a primary care physician for this organizing tool, Peter Roberts MD immediately offered to discuss pertinent issues. His helpful suggestions have enhanced and clarified the text.

Participants in my *Get Organized! Track Your Medical Paperwork* Adult Education classes at Mount St. Mary's College were the first to test out *My Health & Wellness Organizer*. Their positive feedback, encouragement and enthusiasm confirmed that this organizing tool works equally well for those who are healthy but disorganized, those overwhelmed with a health challenge and those who are responsible for helping others—a parent, child, partner or loved one—manage their medical journey.

Thank you one and all!

Dedication

To all those who at some point during treatment have thrown up their hands in exasperation at the mountain of paperwork and thought, "Isn't being sick enough to handle, without all this?"

Introduction to
My Health & Wellness Organizer

Being ill is hard enough without the panic of deciding on doctors and treatment plans or the added stress of record keeping, bills, and filing. Whether you are dealing with an acute or chronic condition or attempting to maintain healthy habits, the need for preparation and organization is the same.

DIS-organization is hazardous to your health! I didn't realize how true that was until I faced my own potentially life-threatening diagnosis. Unprepared for the pressure of making decisions, and constantly accumulating information, I often felt overwhelmed. I even felt that if the illness didn't become my undoing, the paperwork would! I began to create an organizational structure within a three-ring binder to bring myself clarity and sanity.

This easy guide takes the pain out of medical record-keeping.

- No need to try to figure out how to arrange your paperwork. It is all laid out for you.
- Find information when you need it and incorporate new paperwork as it accumulates.
- Become a well-prepared coordinator and manager—even if your medical records are scattered among different doctors.
- It will free your energy and contribute to your sanity—you can more easily focus on your healing.

With clearly defined sections and guidelines for recording your emergency contacts, health history, questions to ask your doctors, tests, treatment, medications, financial & insurance records and resources, *My Health & Wellness Organizer* also helps with decision making, unforeseen medical challenges, end of life issues and much more.

If illness knocks at your door, or at the door of a loved one, you will be prepared!

- *Your mind will NOT go blank when a doctor ask you, "When was the date of your _____ test, or when was the last time you _____?"*
- *You will be able to help a spouse, parent, child or loved one, prepare for medical appointments.*
- *Your loved ones will know where to find your important health information and speak on your behalf when you can't speak for yourself.*
- *You and your whole family will benefit.*

There are many ways to organize your paperwork.
What matters is that <u>you</u> can find everything
—without fuss or stress.

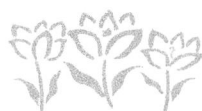

HOW TO ORGANIZE YOUR INFORMATION

Use this 2022 Revision of My Health & Wellness Organizer as your master copy. The author gives you, the purchaser, for your use only, permission to make copies of those pages you will use multiple times. You may then 3-hole punch these "fill-in pages" and insert them into a 3-ring binder ready to add your information when you wish to update your medical journey

Keep It Simple In 6 Steps

1. Fill out the ready-made forms such as "My Yellow Pages" (Pages 5–18)

2. Gather any paperwork you have already accumulated.

3. Sort it out with a support person.

 ✷ Call a friend, family member, colleague or someone you can trust and set a time for this project.

 ✷ Clear and reserve a space on a bookshelf for books and relevant material.

 ✷ Put bulky items, such as articles, magazines and newsletters into folders or magazine boxes, and place them on your shelf along with books.

 ✷ Spread all the remaining papers, (records, reports, notes) out on the top of a table or on the floor to see what you have.

 ✷ Discard any duplicate information.

 ✷ Sort the papers into groups of similar items such as:

   • Notes from conversations with friends

   • Questions for my professional practitioners and their answers

   • Test results

   • Bills, insurance letters and miscellaneous papers

   • Ideas and resources to follow up

 ✷ Clip the papers of each group together.

 ✷ Identify each group by writing its name on a brightly colored slip of paper and put that on the front page of each group.

 ✷ Sort the papers within each group by date or by service provided.

 ✷ Print out additional fill-in pages when you need them.

4. Insert your papers into your *Organizer* binder.

 ✷ Create main sections using the dividers.

 ✷ Punch holes in your papers and insert them in an appropriate section with the most recent on top.

5. Be prepared for your next appointment.
See page 54–57 for helpful ideas and tips.

6. Divide and conquer.

 ✷ Use additional **dividers** to organize your paperwork more precisely so that you can find specific information more easily.

 ✷ Use additional **binders** or one that is much thicker as your papers multiply. For example, treat this as your starter binder, and consider using a separate billing or financial binder.

PART I

MY YELLOW PAGES

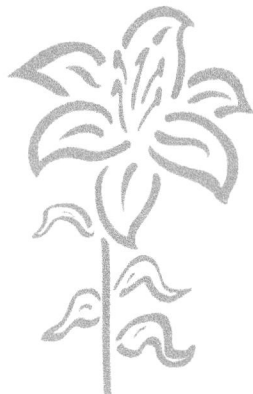

CREATING MY PERSONAL DIRECTORY

Use these pages to record all your most important health-related contacts to create a ready reference directory at your fingertips.

- ❀ **Emergency Contact and Medical Information**

- ❀ **Most Frequently-Used Contacts**
  Make a list of the contact information you expect to refer to constantly. Knowing exactly where to turn for a particular phone number can prevent a lot of unnecessary stress.

- ❀ **Personal Support Team**
  Individuals and Groups

- ❀ **Professional Team**
  Doctors and Other Conventional Health Practitioners
  Complementary, Alternative Medicine (CAM) and Integrative Practitioners

- ❀ **Health Insurance, Legal and Financial Contacts**

- ❀ **Thank you List**—Appreciate help!

- ❀ **Where To Find My Important Papers / Records**—Ease your mind!

AND

- ❀ **Chronological Health History**
  Fill out the log to the best of your ability, including your health history prior to your current diagnosis. Then add your current info: first symptoms [if any] and discovery of your illness, through diagnosis, follow-up tests and results, treatment decisions and all appointments.

  Keep this record of your progress up-to-date. Include any other health concerns. Refer to it during an office visit. You will not have to rack your brain to remember details, and it may prevent you from blanking out, when physicians ask for such information.

  Make sure you continually update these pages.

What matters is that you know where to find everything
—at the drop of a hat!

EMERGENCY CONTACTS AND MEDICAL INFORMATION

Add your emergency telephone contact numbers below and add your primary ICE (In Case of Emergency) numbers to your cell phone contact list.

	NAME	HOME PHONE	CELL PHONE	WORK PHONE
Primary contact:				
If unavailable, contact:				
Next of kin				
Friend				
Walk-In Medical Clinic/ Hospital Emergency Room				
Police, Fire, Ambulance (if in doubt, call 911)				

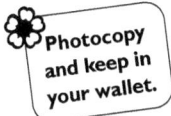

✂

Photocopy and keep in your wallet.

EMERGENCY MEDICAL DATA

Name: _____

Phone: _____

Insurance Co. and ID#: _____

Emergency contact: _____ Phone: _____

Doctor's name: _____ Phone _____

Medical conditions: _____

Medications: _____ Blood group: _____

Medication allergies: _____

- FOLD

Additional information:

_____

_____

_____

_____

_____

_____

_____

_____

_____

MOST FREQUENTLY USED CONTACTS

Put an asterisk * next to the person who is willing to coordinate your treatment.

Name	Telephone / cell	Email

PERSONAL SUPPORT: INDIVIDUALS AND GROUPS

Fill this in after you 1) have made your decisions using the guidelines in Part Two, and 2) have agreement from those whom you have asked. Identify any special role such as a patient navigator or spokesperson for other team members.

INDIVIDUALS (close family, friends, clergy)

Name	Best way to contact - telephone / cell	Email	Address

GROUPS (centers, support groups, organizations)

Name	Best way to contact - telephone / cell	Email	Address

PROFESSIONAL TEAM
MEDICAL DOCTORS AND OTHER CONVENTIONAL HEALTH PRACTITIONERS

Include your primary care doctor, nurse, dentist, eye doctor, and other specialists, such as gynecologist, cardiologist, pediatrician, orthopedist, physical therapist, as you enlist them.

Put an asterisk * next to the person who will coordinate your treatment.

Primary Care Physician _____ My patient # _____

Name of office _____ Insurance accepted YES / NO

Address _____

Tel _____ Other (fax/email/website) _____

Receptionist / secretary _____ Nurse _____

Hospital affiliation _____ Has copy of living will and health care proxy YES / NO

Dentist _____ Specialty _____

Name of office _____ My patient # _____

Address _____ Insurance accepted YES / NO

Tel _____ Other (fax/email/website) _____

Receptionist / secretaryt _____ Nurse / assistant _____

Eye Care Specialist _____ Specialty _____

Name of office _____ My patient # _____

Address _____ Insurance accepted YES / NO

Tel _____ Other (fax/email/website) _____

Receptionist / secretary _____ Nurse / assistant _____

Hospital affiliation _____

Specialist/Second Opinion _____ Specialty _____

Name of office _____ My patient # _____

Address _____ Insurance accepted YES / NO

Tel _____ Other (fax/email/website) _____

Receptionist / secretary _____ Nurse / assistant _____

Hospital affiliation _____

Specialist/Second Opinion _____ Specialty _____

Name of office _____ My patient # _____

Address _____ Insurance accepted YES / NO

Tel _____ Other (fax/email/website) _____

Receptionist / secretary _____ Nurse / assistant _____

Hospital affiliation _____

PROFESSIONAL TEAM
COMPLEMENTARY, ALTERNATIVE AND INTEGRATIVE MEDICAL PRACTITIONERS

Include your holistic doctor, nurse, acupuncturist, naturopath, healer, massage therapist, chiropractor, cranial-sacral body worker, counselor and/or others.

Put an asterisk * next to the person who is willing to coordinate your medical care.

Name_____ My patient #_____

Modality _____

Name of office _____ Insurance accepted YES / NO

Address_____

Tel _____ Other (fax/email/website) _____

Receptionist / secretary_____ Nurse_____

Hospital affiliation_____ Has copy of living will and health care proxy YES / NO

Name_____ My patient #_____

Modality _____

Name of office _____ Insurance accepted YES / NO

Address_____

Tel _____ Other (fax/email/website) _____

Receptionist / secretary_____ Nurse_____

Hospital affiliation_____ Has copy of living will and health care proxy YES / NO

Name_____ My patient #_____

Modality _____

Name of office _____ Insurance accepted YES / NO

Address_____

Tel _____ Other (fax/email/website) _____

Receptionist / secretary_____ Nurse_____

Hospital affiliation_____ Has copy of living will and health care proxy YES / NO

Name_____ My patient #_____

Modality _____

Name of office _____ Insurance accepted YES / NO

Address_____

Tel _____ Other (fax/email/website) _____

Receptionist / secretary_____ Nurse_____

Hospital affiliation_____ Has copy of living will and health care proxy YES / NO

PROFESSIONAL TEAM
INSURANCE, LEGAL, AND FINANCIAL CONTACTS

HEALTH INSURANCE

Primary health insurance company _____

Membership ID _____ Effective date _____

Plan name _____Policy/group number _____

Contact person_____Tel/fax/email _____

Secondary health insurance company _____

Membership ID _____ Effective date _____

Plan name _____Policy/group number _____

Contact person_____Tel/fax/email _____

Other Insurance, such as long-term care_____

Membership ID _____ Effective date _____

Plan name _____Policy/group number _____

Contact person_____Tel/fax/email _____

LEGAL

Healthcare proxy_____

Address_____

Tel/fax/email _____

Relationship _____ Has copy of my living will and healthcare proxy form   YES / NO

Lawyer _____

Address_____ Secretary/assistant_____

Tel/fax/email _____

Has copy of my will, living will and healthcare proxy form   YES / NO

Power of attorney _____

Address_____

Tel/fax/email _____

Relationship _____ Has copy of my will, living will and healthcare proxy form   YES / NO

Back-up contact (Health Proxy / Power of Attorney)_____

Tel/ email _____

Realtionship _____

PROFESSIONAL TEAM
INSURANCE, LEGAL, AND FINANCIAL CONTACTS (cont'd)

Additional people (e.g. family members, doctors) who have a copy of my legal papers

Name	Will	Living will	Healthcare proxy
_____	☐	☐	☐
_____	☐	☐	☐
_____	☐	☐	☐
_____	☐	☐	☐
_____	☐	☐	☐

FINANCIAL

Financial advisor _____ Tel _____

Office address_____

Secretary/assistant _____Tel _____

Fax_____ Email_____ Cell _____

Tax Preparer/accountant _____

Office address_____

Secretary/assistant _____Tel _____

Fax_____ Email_____ Cell _____

Bank _____ Bank manager _____

Branch address _____

Branch tel _____Customer service tel _____

Online banking info_____

Other _____

Address_____

Best contact info. _____

THANK YOU LIST

Here you can keep a record of any gifts of love, or kind thoughtful actions, no matter how small, as well as when and how you have expressed your gratitude.

Person to thank + contact info	For call / card / email	Thanked by date

WHERE TO FIND MY IMPORTANT PAPERS / RECORDS

For ease of mind, list where you keep all your important information. Once completed, provide a copy for your lawyer and close family members. LAST UPDATED:_____

Item	Located in						
	Bank safety deposit bo x	Home firebox	Home filing cabinet	Office	Lawyer's office	Wallet	Other
Computer Passwords							
Back up drive							
Financial							
Bank accounts							
Credit card info.							
IOUs							
IRAs / Roths							
Investments							
Retirement and pension							
Tax returns							
Other							
House / Home							
Deed / Mortgage							
Rental							
Other							
Insurance							
Car (+ title, registration)							
Health							
House / rental							
Other							
Legal							
Healthcare proxy							
Living will							
Organ donor info.							
Power of Attorney							
Will / Trust							
Other							
Personal							
Birth certificate							
Divorce/separation papers							
Driver's license							
Funeral arrangements							
Marriage certificate							
Passport							
Social Security Number							
Other							

CURRENT CHRONOLOGICAL HEALTH HISTORY

Create an overview of your current general medical information to the best of your ability. You will be able to give a copy to all your health care providers when they request it.

GENERAL MEDICAL INFORMATION

Today's date (mm / dd / yyyy) _____

Name _____ Age _____ Date of birth _____

Street _____City _____State _____ Zip _____

Home tel _____ Cell tel; _____ Work tel _____

Blood type _____ Social Security # _____

Next of kin / emergency contact _____ Best way to reach _____

Health Care Proxy _____ Best way to reach_____

Allergies (with medications, if any) _____

Vital signs, recorded by staff before you meet a doctor:

Date	Weight	Height	Blood Pressure	Pulse
_____	_____	_____	_____	_____
_____	_____	_____	_____	_____
_____	_____	_____	_____	_____
_____	_____	_____	_____	_____
_____	_____	_____	_____	_____

Previous surgeries, if any, with dates_____

_____

Other medical conditions and medications _____

_____

Any other information you think is important_____

_____

PAST / CURRENT FAMILY HISTORY

List significant illness(es) and / or cause of death for immediate family members:

Mother _____

Father _____

Siblings _____

CURRENT CHRONOLOGICAL HEALTH HISTORY (cont'd)

SOCIAL & HEALTH HISTORY

Occupation _____

Marital status _____

Please list the amount consumed:

Alcoholic beverages per day _____ /week _____ Cigarettes per day _____ /week_____

Glasses of soda per day _____ / week _____ How often do you exercise per week? _____times

How many hours sleep do you generally get per night? _____ hours

Do you wear your seat belt regularly?   Yes   No

Have you experienced problems with any of the following? If yes, please explain below.

Heart / Vascular	☐ no	☐ yes*
Breathing	☐ no	☐ yes
Stomach / Intestines	☐ no	☐ yes
Female / Male Organs	☐ no	☐ yes
Kidney / Bladder	☐ no	☐ yes
Brain / Spinal Cord	☐ no	☐ yes
Muscles / Joints / Bone	☐ no	☐ yes
Thyroid	☐ no	☐ yes
Skin	☐ no	☐ yes
Cancerous Growths	☐ no	☐ yes

*Explanation of any of the above: _____

_____

_____

_____

CURRENT HEALTH CHALLENGE

Chief complaint: _____

When did you first notice something was wrong? _____

What did you experience? _____

Circle severity of pain on scale   1   2   3   4   5   6   7   8   9   10

(1 = hardly noticeable and 10 = most severe)

Other Comments_____

_____

_____

CHRONOLOGICAL HEALTH HISTORY (cont'd)

DIAGNOSIS given for current health challenge _____

Given by _____ Date (mm/dd/yyyy) _____

Facility _____

Doctor's follow-up recommendations _____

My response _____

Additional consultations, 2nd opinions and tests to help me decide my treatment

Health Professional _____ Date _____

    Facility _____

    Purpose _____

    Findings/recommendations _____

    _____ Reports / tests filed under _____

Health Professional _____ Date _____

    Facility _____

    Purpose _____

    Findings/recommendations _____

    _____ Reports / tests filed under _____

Health Professional _____ Date _____

    Facility _____

    Purpose _____

    Findings/recommendations _____

    _____ Reports / tests filed under _____

Health Professional _____ Date _____

    Facility _____

    Purpose _____

    Findings/recommendations _____

    _____ Reports / tests filed under _____

CHRONOLOGICAL HEALTH HISTORY (cont'd)

MY CURRENT TREATMENT DECISION(S) _____ Date (mm/dd/yyyy) _____

E.g. Surgery, physical therapy, medication, diet, naturopathy, radiation, acupuncture, counseling, chiropractic, etc.

Remember to review PART 2 before making ANY decisions!

FIRST TREATMENT Date _____ Location _____

With _____ or under the supervision of _____

Treatment / tests given _____ Reports / tests filed under_____

Medication(s) prescribed _____

Notes _____

FURTHER TREATMENTS / APPOINTMENTS

Add all consultations, tests and test results, adjuvant therapies, alternative therapies, drugs, and prescribed medications in chronological order under the headings below:

Date _____ Reason for visit _____

With _____ or under the supervision of _____

Treatment / tests given _____ Reports / tests filed under_____

Medication(s) prescribed _____

Notes _____

Date _____ Reason for visit _____

With _____ or under the supervision of _____

Treatment / tests given _____ Reports / tests filed under_____

Medication(s) prescribed _____

Notes _____

Date _____ Reason for visit _____

With _____ or under the supervision of _____

Treatment / tests given _____ Reports / tests filed under_____

Medication(s) prescribed _____

Notes _____

CHRONOLOGICAL HEALTH HISTORY (cont'd)

FURTHER TREATMENTS / APPOINTMENTS

Date _____ Reason for visit_____

With _____ or under the supervision of_____

Treatment / tests given _____ Reports / tests filed under _____

Medication(s) prescribed _____

Notes _____

Date _____ Reason for visit_____

With _____ or under the supervision of_____

Treatment / tests given _____ Reports / tests filed under _____

Medication(s) prescribed _____

Notes _____

Date _____ Reason for visit_____

With _____ or under the supervision of_____

Treatment / tests given _____ Reports / tests filed under _____

Medication(s) prescribed _____

Notes _____

Date _____ Reason for visit_____

With _____ or under the supervision of_____

Treatment / tests given _____ Reports / tests filed under _____

Medication(s) prescribed _____

Notes _____

Date _____ Reason for visit_____

With _____ or under the supervision of_____

Treatment / tests given _____ Reports / tests filed under _____

Medication(s) prescribed _____

Notes _____

PART 2

DECISIONS, DECISIONS, DECISIONS

MAKE PERSONAL SUPPORT DECISIONS

You may not initially know if you need help or what your needs will be or even how to ask for help and from whom, but when you do...

USE THE QUESTIONS on the following pages to help you clarify the kind of support you wish to have.

Ask yourself how you'd like your family, friends and community to support you with specific tasks. (These may be different from what people offer you). It's important to identify the help you *do* need and make your decisions. You can gently refuse help you do not need. List those whom you wish to ask.

TAKE ACTION

- Invite those you have chosen to help you.

- Ask for what you need; this is not a time to go it alone.

- Delegate.

- Add the contact information of those who have agreed to be on your "*Personal Support Team*" on page 7 in *My Yellow Pages*. (Remember that too many people can be overwhelming, and it can be helpful to choose a spokesperson).

UPDATE FROM TIME TO TIME

- Review *My Personal Wellness Commitments* on page 51.

A FEW PRETTY GOOD TIPS

WHEN MAKING DECISIONS

Following the shock of your diagnosis, you may be in turmoil and not know how best to make decisions.

✳ VERY IMPORTANT!
This is a perfect time to reach out to the trusted people in your life, be they family, friends, professionals, a person who has experienced your health problem or navigator to help you handle these challenging issues and daunting questions. This is not a time to go it alone.

❀ It is important to clarify your preferences by noting both your thoughts and feelings *before* you make any decisions.

❀ *Please take your time.*

❀ Give yourself a break between each question.

❀ Ask your helper to go through it with you, and if it is easier for you, ask him or her to make a note of your answers.

If this feels overwhelming to you, just do what you can.

WHAT ARE MY NEEDS AT THIS TIME?

What practical support would I most appreciate?
E.g. Errands, child care, special food, driving to appointments?

What emotional support would I most appreciate?
E.g. Call after appointments, listen, help me look at options?

What spiritual support would I most appreciate?
E.g. Set up prayer circle, inspirational readings, walk with friend, connect with spiritual mentor?

What would NOT be of help to me?
E.g. Constant invasive phone questions, lasagna (if that's not a food I like)?

How can I best ask for what I do need?
E.g. Be honest with self, and then with others?

HOW CAN FAMILY AND FRIENDS HELP ME MEET THESE NEEDS?

What are the strengths of my close family members and friends?

Who   What

_____

_____

_____

_____

Who is good at doing what?

Who   What

_____

_____

_____

_____

What have my family members and friends offered to do, if anything?

Who   What

_____

_____

_____

_____

How would I like them to be involved?

Who   What

_____

_____

_____

_____

Would I benefit from having someone in a special role such as spokesperson, to pass on information to other team members? If so, how?

WHAT OTHER COMMUNITY SUPPORT WOULD BE HELPFUL TO ME?

Support / patient group

Religious / spiritual organization

Internet

Blog

Social network

Chat group

Other...

HOW WOULD I LIKE OTHERS TO HELP ME?

Prioritize and list your needs.

Make a couple of copies: one to put on the fridge or beside your phone and one to carry with you, so you won't draw a blank when you are asked what help you need.

Help I need	When? now or later / date	Person I'll ask / who offered	Date completed

MY PERSONAL SUPPORT TEAM

List those special people you wish to invite to be members of your personal support team.

Add their contact information to *My Personal Support Team* page in *My Yellow Pages*, when they have agreed. *Remember to identify your spokesperson, if you have one.

Name	Phone #	Date invited	To help with	Now/later

MAKE TREATMENT DECISIONS AND ENLIST PROFESSIONAL SUPPORT

Decide initial treatment preferences
Refine treatment choices
Sharpen focus towards a more considered opinion
Finalize treatment decisions
Choose professional team

If you have already agreed to a treatment plan, or your feel this section does not apply to you, please SKIP it for now and move the pages of this section to the back of your binder.

TAKE ACTION

Identify and invite the professionals whom you wish to be responsible for the treatments you have chosen.

Add the contact information for each to your Yellow Pages, when they have agreed.

Ask yourself, **"Who will coordinate my treatment?"**

> This person will oversee your total treatment plan. Your primary physician is often the most appropriate choice. Choose someone you are comfortable with. If that person is not able to do so, ask for another referral.

The person who has agreed to coordinate my treatment is

Name: Best way to contact:

If you can't find such a willing person, use your *Health & Wellness Organizer*, with your notes and your questions, as a resource to help you be your own overseer—and your own advocate.

Take your binder to appointments as a reminder that your medical care can be a coordinated service.

A FEW PRETTY GOOD TIPS

TAKE YOUR TIME

It is important to clarify your preferences by noting both your thoughts and feelings before you make any treatment decisions or enlist the support of any practitioner. However, please take your time. Hasty decisions may not be in your best interests. If this thorough approach feels overwhelming to you, just do what you can.

⊛ Give yourself a break between the steps that follow.

⊛ Ask a friend or family member to go through it with you, and perhaps make a note of your answers.

⊛ Do whatever feels useful to you in order to be ready to select your treatment and professional team…and leave the rest.

WHAT DO I PREFER?
DECIDE INITIAL TREATMENT PREFERENCES

1. What kinds of diagnostic tools and interventions have worked for me in the past?

2. For my specific diagnosis, what do I see to be the benefits and strengths of:

- Conventional medicine?

- Complementary and alternative care?

- A combination of conventional and complementary modalities or an integrative approach by a medical doctor who has been trained in both?

3. How confident, comfortable, and hopeful do I feel treating my medical issue(s) with recommendations and prescriptions of:

- Conventional physicians?

- Complementary and alternative care practitioners?

- Integrative practitioners?

REFINE TREATMENT CHOICES

Use the following charts to further clarify your initial treatment preferences by checking the appropriate box below.

Conventional Options

TESTS

	YES I'm comfortable using this test	NO I'm not interested	DON'T KNOW I want more info
Biopsy	☐	☐	☐
Blood sample analysis	☐	☐	☐
CAT scan or CT scan	☐	☐	☐
Genetic Testing	☐	☐	☐
Mammography	☐	☐	☐
MRI	☐	☐	☐
Palpating	☐	☐	☐
PET scan	☐	☐	☐
Radiographic studies (X-ray)	☐	☐	☐
Ultrasound	☐	☐	☐
Others (such as colonoscopy, heart stress test)			
_____	☐	☐	☐
_____	☐	☐	☐

TREATMENTS

	YES I'm comfortable using this test	NO I'm not interested	DON'T KNOW I want more info
Bed rest	☐	☐	☐
Biopsy	☐	☐	☐
Chemotherapy	☐	☐	☐
Diet	☐	☐	☐
Exercise	☐	☐	☐
Immunotherapy	☐	☐	☐
Medication	☐	☐	☐
Physical therapy	☐	☐	☐
Other_____	☐	☐	☐
_____	☐	☐	☐

REFINE TREATMENT CHOICES (cont'd)
Complementary Options
TESTS

	YES I'm comfortable using this test	NO I'm not interested	DON'T KNOW I want more info
Biofeedback	☐	☐	☐
Detailed life history	☐	☐	☐
Eye, tongue and skin exam	☐	☐	☐
Genetic testing	☐	☐	☐
Muscle testing	☐	☐	☐
Pulses	☐	☐	☐
Thermography	☐	☐	☐
Other_____	☐	☐	☐

TREATMENTS

	YES I'm comfortable using this test	NO I'm not interested	DON'T KNOW I want more info
Acupuncture	☐	☐	☐
Aromatherapy	☐	☐	☐
Ayurvedic	☐	☐	☐
Bach flower essences	☐	☐	☐
Biofeedback	☐	☐	☐
Chiropractic	☐	☐	☐
Energy healing	☐	☐	☐
Essential oils	☐	☐	☐
Health kinesiology	☐	☐	☐
Holistic nursing	☐	☐	☐
Homeopathy	☐	☐	☐
Massage therapy	☐	☐	☐
Meditation	☐	☐	☐
Mental health counseling	☐	☐	☐
Naturopathy	☐	☐	☐
Nutritional / herbal counseling	☐	☐	☐
Osteopathic manipulation	☐	☐	☐
Physical therapy	☐	☐	☐
Reflexology	☐	☐	☐
Spiritual healing	☐	☐	☐
Tai Chi	☐	☐	☐
Traditional Chinese medicine	☐	☐	☐
Yoga	☐	☐	☐
Other _____	☐	☐	☐

SHARPEN FOCUS TOWARDS A MORE CONSIDERED OPINION

1. **Add up all the times you checked YES. Note where most are on your chart.**

    Number of YES checks for conventional treatment_____
    Number of YES checks for complementary/alternative treatment_____

2. **Consider all the information you have thus far gained from your experience, discussions and research, and ask:**

    Given the type and severity of my condition, what are my reasons for:

    *   choosing conventional treatments?

    *   choosing complementary and/or alternative treatments?

    *   choosing to integrate conventional and complementary treatments?

3. **Ask, "What else would I like to know before making a fully informed choice?"**

    For example, do I need to ask more questions such as:

    *   What is the advice of my physician and/or my complementary and alternative medicine (CAM) health provider?

    *   Have I been given any choices of treatment? If not, ask to initiate that discussion.

    *   What conventional treatments have been specifically recommended for my condition?

    *   What complementary/alternative treatments have been specifically recommended?

    *   What treatments are congruent with my perspectives about healing?

    *   What is the evidence in support of all these specific recommendations?

    *   What do clinical trials, if any, of patients with my type and stage of illness show about such treatments?

4. **Tap into your intuition**

    I will take time to slow down, e.g. by walking in nature, so that I can feel my inner response to each possibility, and ask, "What is my gut feeling now about each approach?"

SHARPEN FOCUS TOWARDS A MORE CONSIDERED OPINION (cont'd)

If I need further information about a specific question or concern noted on the previous page, I will call on the appropriate resource/person to help me get the pertinent information.

Issue / question	Possible resource	Person to ask for assistance
	Library The internet Organizations Local support groups Other _____	
	Library The internet Organizations Local support groups Other _____	
	Library The internet Organizations Local support groups Other _____	
	Library The internet Organizations Local support groups Other _____	

Research notes

FINALIZE TREATMENT DECISIONS

❧ **What is my considered judgment now about what would help my body heal...**

...from conventional medicine?

...from complementary care?

...from alternative care?

❧ **Does this feel right to me?**

❧ **I now choose the following modalities for treatment:**

Initially:

Along with:

Followed by:

CHOOSING MY PROFESSIONAL TEAM

HEALTH PROFESSIONALS WHO ARE ALREADY ON MY TEAM:

Name of physician or health professional	**Area of expertise**

ADDITIONAL PROFESSIONAL SUPPORT I NEED

Ask yourself, "What other specialists or professional skills do I need for my healing"?

Identify the support you need, ask for recommendations and leads, and then list below those you wish to follow up: (e.g. an internist? an acupuncturist?)

Area of expertise	**Physician or health professional suggested**	**Recommended by**

FOR EACH SPECIALIST, ASK, "WHAT CRITERIA IS MOST IMPORTANT TO ME?"

	Very important	Important	Not a concern
Training and qualifications*			
Professional reputation and peer reviews			
Distance—how far am I willing to travel?			
Openness to communicate with other professionals			
Ability to listen to my questions and communicate clearly			
Staff and facility welcoming and approachable			
Other (For example, will my insurance be accepted?)			

Make sure any physician is "Board Certified" in their specialty

CHOOSING MY PROFESSIONAL TEAM (Cont'd)

Record the results of your inquiries. Then note your decision whether to continue with each practitioner.

Name	Specialty	Date contacted	By phone or in person	Decided to follow up: YES / NO

✺ **If you feel hopeful, supported and compatible with a practitioner you've contacted, and you are ready to follow up with this practitioner, invite them to become a member of your professional team. Then add his or her contact information to your Professional List in** *My Yellow Pages.*

PART 3

MY MEDICAL APPOINTMENTS

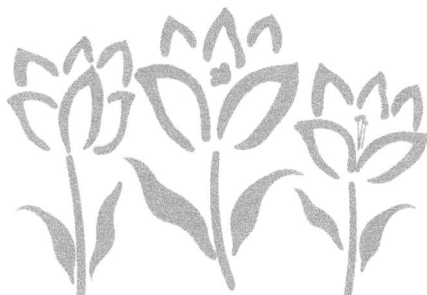

MAKING THE MOST OF MY MEDICAL APPOINTMENTS

Part 3 My Medical Appointments **offers four sets of questions that you might ask in different circumstances, all adaptable to your own situation.**

> **Introductory questions** to ask at your annual physical check-up or when you don't feel well. (Pages 37–38))

> **More detailed questions** to ask when a practitioner gives a diagnosis or recommends tests, treatment, or seeing a specialist. (Pages 39–45)

> **Examples of questions specifically targeted** to two different kinds of specialists: a heart-cardiovascular specialist and an orthopedist. (Pages 46–49) These can also be adapted to your specific illness. (For cancer-related concerns and questions, *My Hope & Focus Cancer Organizer* would be appropriate. For information, see www.rootsnwings.com.)

> **Questions for any practitioner** about keeping your lifestyle healthy and when you are nearing the end of treatment. (Pages 50–53)

BEFORE ANY MEDICAL APPOINTMENT

Whether about a diagnosis, treatment or test, ask yourself, **"What do I want to know?"**

> **Highlight** the questions listed on the following pages that you wish to ask. Cross out those you do not wish to ask and add any others. Adapt the questions for your situation, always using words that come naturally to you.

AT YOUR IN-PERSON OR TELEMEDICINE VISIT

Ask the doctor your questions, and if allowed, ask your companion / navigator to note the answers.

A FEW PRETTY GOOD TIPS

PREPARE DETAILED QUESTIONS IN ADVANCE

This will help you to get the most out of your medical visits:

❋ Plan ahead to invite a member of your personal support team or a local advocacy group to go with you, if post-Covid mandates allow this. Otherwise ask permission to record specific info.

❋ Review, reorder and regroup your questions / concerns in your own words on the following pages or on a new sheet of paper.

❋ Go through the list systematically to make sure that you have nothing left to check or if the wording could be more precise. It's your right to have your questions answered, but physicians are very busy people. Be as succinct and clear as possible. If your questions are clear, your doctors' answers can be more focused and helpful.

❋ Make extra copies of the list to take with you, one for the person accompanying you and one for your physician or health professional, if you wish him or her to have it.

❋ Respect the limits of what you can comfortably handle at any one time as you do this preparation. Take breaks and enlist help so that you don't get overwhelmed. While it is normal to feel overwhelmed, being well prepared will build your confidence.

QUESTIONS for...

MY PRIMARY CARE PHYSICIAN
AT MY ANNUAL ROUTINE PHYSICAL EXAMINATION

Dr. _____ Date (mmddyyyy)_____

1. Expect a nurse or staff member to take your blood pressure, pulse and ask you to give a urine sample before you see the doctor. If asked, fill out or update your health history profile on your doctor's form. (refer to your health history log on pages 14–15)

2. Expect your doctor to ask you the following questions, especially if you are a new patient. (It is likely that you will have prepared answers to these questions in your chronological health history on pages 14–15.)

  a. Have you noticed any changes since your last visit?

     What is your past medical history?

     Do you have any allergies?

     Family medical history

  b. List all medications are you taking. Any new medications?

  c. What is your activity level?   Per day/week/month

       Walking

       Sports

       Other

  d. What is your alcohol, tobacco and drug use? (Please list)

  e. Any recent visits to any other doctors? (E.g. cardiologist, or other specialist) If my office does not have these results/reports, please request that they be sent in the future.

3. Be prepared to ask these questions:

  a. What is my blood pressure?

  b. What was the result of my urine analysis?

  c. What suggestions do you have for me to maintain and improve my health?

  d. Do you recommend any tests? If so, what are they, and why are they needed?

  e. Given my health history, should I have any adult immunizations? (For example: Tetanus shot, Flu shot, other)

  f. What are your specific recommendations regarding next steps?

NOTE: Your primary care physician's questions will also be similar to those *any* health professional will ask you on a first visit—whatever your medical issue may be.

Being prepared to answer or ask these questions will come in handy at other health visits.

QUESTIONS for...

MY DOCTOR WHEN I DON'T FEEL WELL
AND WANT TO KNOW WHAT'S WRONG

Adapt this page for your dentist, eye care specialist, audiologist, chiropractor and others.

Dr. _____ Date (mmddyyyy) _____

1. Expect your doctor to ask you the following questions and be prepared to answer them as clearly as you can:

a. What's the problem / why did you make this appointment?

b. What is your chief complaint—the **single** most important symptom? Focus on the immediate problem and avoid bringing in other symptoms, until the doctor asks you.

c. Tell me the "history" of your current complaint:

How long have you been experiencing symptoms?

What was the onset like—gradual / sudden?

Did you notice any precipitating factors?

How do you experience your pain—sharp / dull / throbbing / numb / etc.? Where in your body do you feel this pain?

How often do you experience this—recurrent / daily / night?

Progress—better / worse / unchanged?

Have you done anything to alleviate your pain? If so, what have you done? Has it helped?

2. Make sure your doctor answers these questions before you end your appointment.

Q: What is wrong with me? Can you give me a diagnosis?
A:

Q: What treatment do you recommend? Now? Later?
A:

Q: What should I do if symptoms worsen?
A:

Q: Should I have a follow up appointment? With you? With a specialist? With a health practitioner trained in a different modality?
A:

3. Ask your physician to repeat any instructions.

IN AN EMERGENCY, WHEN YOUR DOCTOR IS NOT AVAILABLE, CONTACT THE WALK-IN CLINIC OR HOSPITAL EMERGENCY FACILITY YOU HAVE LISTED ON PAGE 5

QUESTIONS
about...

MY DIAGNOSIS

Dr. _____ Date (mmddyyyy) _____

Q: What's wrong with me? What exactly is my diagnosis?
A:

Q: Please describe my condition in simple language?
A:

Q: How did you arrive at your opinion? How certain are you? Is there a test to confirm this diagnosis?
A:

Q: What symptoms have you observed or have I reported to you that led to your diagnosis?
A:

Q: Could there be other reasons for my symptoms?
A:

Q: Can a test can confirm my diagnosis?
A:

Q: How will this diagnosis affect my life? ie. Which daily activities are okay, and which must I avoid?
A:

Q: How serious is this? Can my illness go into remission? What is your definition of remission?
   Disease-free for 5 or _____ years? How will I know if I am in remission?
A:

Q: What about a cure? How will I know if I am cured? For how long can I expect to be disease-free?
   (For 3–5 years, or the rest of my life, or what?)
A:

Q: What must I now take into consideration? Do I need to be alert to symptoms in any other part of
   my body?
A:

Q: What do we need to do next?
A:

QUESTIONS
for...   A DOCTOR WHO SUGGESTS A MEDICAL TEST

Dr. _____ Date (mmddyyyy) _____

Consider these questions when your health professional recommends a test such as a stress test, throat swab, comprehensive metabolic panel, Vitamin D level, mammogram, biopsy, ultrasound, MRI, X-RAY, CT Scan, PET scan, a scope (colonoscopy/bronchoscopy) or lab work such as CBC (complete blood count), thermography.

Q: What test(s) or lab work are you recommending?
A:

Q: What do you hope to find out? What is the purpose of the test(s)?
A:

Q: Will this test confirm a diagnosis you have already given me or about which you are unsure? How will it help you (the doctor) or me come to a more informed decision?
A:

Q: May I take the test in your office? Now? If later, when, where and with whom?
A:

Q: What will the procedure entail? (Please describe the length of time it will take, requirements to be immobile, etc.)
A:

Q: Do I need to fast before this test?
A:

Q: When will I get results? How will I find out?
A:

Footnote to myself (and to discuss with a support person)

Q: If a conventional doctor is recommending a test, do I want or need any second opinions or a different viewpoint?
A:

Q: If a complementary practitioner is recommending a test, have I checked to make sure I won't be duplicating a test ordered by my conventional medicine doctor?
A:

✂ **Ask that copies of any test results be sent directly to yourself as well as to the doctor.**

QUESTIONS about...

MY TEST RESULTS

Dr. _____ Date (mmddyyyy) _____

Use this page when you are given any test results.

Test given	Date of test	Location of test

Q: What do these results mean?

A:

Q: What new information do you have?

A:

Q: If my results are coded in numbers, what do the numbers mean?

A:

Q: Are my numbers within the normal range _____? Higher than normal_____? Lower than normal _____? What is considered within the normal range for this test?

A:

Q: If this is a repeat test, are there any changes? If so, what are they and what do they mean for me?

A:

Q: Do you recommend regular testing and/or any additional tests? If so, what, where, and how often?

A:

Q: Given the results of this test and your experience with this disease, how serious is my condition? Is it life-threatening? Be truthful, please. (I understand that no one can predict exactly what any outcome will be, nor can statistics.)

A:

❧ **Remember to ask for copies of test results before you leave the office.**

QUESTIONS about...

MY TREATMENT OPTIONS

Dr. _____ Date (mmddyyyy) _____

Q: What are my treatment options?
A:

Q: Which of these are standard treatments? And with which have you had success?
A:

Q: Are there alternatives? If so, what are they?
A:

Q: For each possible option, please tell me where the treatment will be given, how long it will last and how often it will be given.
A:

Q: What are the **benefits** of this treatment?   Short-term?   Long-term?
A:

Q: What are the **risks** of this treatment?   Short-term?   Long-term?
A:

Q: What are the **side effects** of this treatment?   Short-term?   Long-term?
A:

Q: Where can I learn more about this treatment _____ for my condition?
A:

Q: Do you know of any experimental treatments or clinical trials for my kind of illness that you would recommend for me?
A:

Q: I know you can't see into the future, but from your medical training what is the likely course of events if I do nothing?
A:

Q: Is it better to get a second opinion now before anything is done, or wait till after the tests, surgery or other procedures that you may be recommending? Why?
A:

❧ **Question for myself** (to discuss with a support person):
Q: Do I have enough information? If not, what is lacking?
A:

QUESTIONS about... MY DOCTOR'S TREATMENT RECOMMENDATIONS

Dr. _____ Date (mmddyyyy) _____

Select the questions you would like to ask when your doctor recommends a specific treatment such as surgery, bed-rest, exercise, medication, transplant, chemotherapy, hormonal therapy, physical therapy, massage, dialysis, injections, hypnotherapy, diet, counseling or anything else:

Q: What are your specific recommendations?
A:

Q: What are your reasons for recommending _____?
A:

Q: How did you decide which treatment(s) to recommend to me?
A:

Q: If you are recommending medication, what drugs will be used, and for how long?

A: **Name of drug**	**Benefits**	**Potential side effects**

Q: Are there any foods I should or should not eat during treatment? What about alcohol? Smoking? Vitamins?
A:

Q: If surgery is recommended, how soon can I bend/lift/drive/take part in sports/exercise? What exercises should I do or avoid?
A:

Q: How will I know if the treatments are working/not working?
A:

Q: Who will monitor my progress? How? Whom may I consult if I experience any problems?
A:

Q: Can you show me research that would give me confidence in the specific intervention(s) you are recommending?
A:

QUESTIONS about...

TIMING OF RECOMMENDED TREATMENTS

Dr. _____ Date (mmddyyyy) _____

Q: What treatment decisions do you recommend I must make NOW—before I leave your office or within 24-48 hours? If so, is this because you consider my diagnosis to be life-threatening?

A:

Q: What decisions must I make SOON? How soon?

A:

Q: What decisions can I make LATER?

A:

Q: How long may I wait before deciding on my choices?

A:

Q: If you are recommending a later decision, why is that?

A:

Q: Does a specific treatment have to come after or before another treatment?

A:

Q: What amount of "wiggle-room" do I have to do further research, without being pressured by fear or time constraints?

A:

Q: How long is the treatment? And how lengthy is the recuperation?

A:

Questions for myself (and discuss with a support person)

Q: If a physician is recommending immediate treatment within a few days, do I understand, and agree with, this urgency as a medical necessity?

A:

Q: Have I had enough time to absorb the shock and make peace with my decision?

A:

Q: Do I need more information before deciding? If so, what and from whom?

A:

QUESTIONS for...

MY COMPLEMENTARY, ALTERNATIVE
AND INTEGRATIVE PRACTITIONERS

Dr. _____ Date (mmddyyyy) _____

Tell the specialist or practitioner clearly why you are seeking help:

☐ To complement your conventional physicians

☐ Specifically for pain management or nausea

☐ For a general consultation

☐ For an alternative approach, complete in itself. (See treatments listed on page 29.)

Check above or add your reason here:

_____

Q: What can I expect from your approach?

A:

Q: How much experience have you had with _____ patients and conventional treatments for my disease?

A:

Q: Are you willing to work with Western conventional doctors?

A:

Q: What is the knowledge base for the treatment you are recommending? Specifically, is there any research about the course of action you are asking me to take?

A:

Q: What are the benefits and risks of this treatment?

A:

Q: What is the length of treatment?

A:

Q: If you are suggesting vitamins and supplements please specify brand names you know to be trustworthy and tell me why you are recommending them.

A:

Q: How will your suggestions for diet, whole food and supplements affect my conventional treatment?

A:

Q: What out-of-pocket costs will be involved? Fees for each visit? For supplements, etc?

A:

QUESTIONS
for...   A HEART AND CARDIOVASCULAR SPECIALIST

Dr. _____ Date (mmddyyyy) _____

Use these two pages when you have been referred to, or have chosen to consult, a cardiologist because of concerns with your heart; for example, if you experience symptoms such as: irregular pulse or heart beat, edema of the legs, problems with a heart valve, heart murmur or high blood pressure.

BEFORE A DIAGNOSIS, describe your concerns:

I have the following symptoms: chest pain, shortness of breath, pain or numbness in

my_____ and /or elsewhe

re_____

My level of pain on a scale of 1(minor) to 10 (intense) is (circle one):

1   2   3   4   5   6   7   8   9   10

Be prepared to ask questions such as:

Q: Do I have a heart or cardiovascular problem? If so, what is it?
A:

Q: I have a family history of heart disease; how might that affect my health?
A:

Q: If my condition is not hereditary, what can I do to take care of my health now?
A:

Q: Do you advise a stress test / cardiovascular evaluation?
A:

Q: Do I need a follow-up to my treadmill stress test, such as nuclear stress test?
A:

Q: What can I do to prevent a heart attack or other heart problems?
A:

Refer also to the questions about *Keeping My Lifestyle Healthy* on pages 50–51 such as:

Q: How can I reduce my stress and anxiety?
A:

QUESTIONS
for...   A HEART AND CARDIOVASCULAR SPECIALIST (cont'd.)

AFTER RECEIVING A DIAGNOSIS (Following test results)

Q: What is wrong with my heart? What form of heart or cardiovascular disease do I have?

A:

Q: How severe is my heart condition? What is my prognosis?

A:

Q: What are my treatment options? Surgery? Medication? Other?

A:

Q: What should I do if my heart disease symptoms suddenly get worse?

A:

Q: How will you or I know if I need further tests or treatment?

A:

Q: Should I be concerned about high blood pressure (hypertension)? Do I need to lower my blood pressure? If so, how?

A:

Q: What role does cholesterol play in heart and cardiovascular disease? Do I have high cholesterol? Do I need to lower my cholesterol? If so, how?

A:

Q: What are the risks of not treating my heart or cardiovascular problem?

A:

Q: Should I enroll in a cardiac rehabilitation program to strengthen my heart?

A:

Q: Am I eligible for any clinical trials?

A:

Q: How will my diagnosis affect daily activities, such as lifting, having sex, playing sports?

A:

QUESTIONS for...

AN ORTHOPEDIST
Specializing in muscle, joint, ligament and bone problems,
connected to the feet, ankles, legs, hips, or to the shoulders, arms, wrists and hands.

Dr. _____ Date (mmddyyyy) _____

BEFORE A DIAGNOSIS

Be prepared to describe your condition (reason for visit):

I am most concerned about_____

_____

Cause, if known:

   Result of an injury / accident _____

   Result of conditions at work such as repetitive movement_____

   Other? _____

My level of pain on a scale of 1(minor) to 10 (intense) is (circle one): **1   2   3   4   5   6   7   8   9   10**

I most often experience the sensation of pain as: sharp / dull / hot / throbbing / numb / other_____

My mobility, or range of motion, is limited as follows: _____

WHEN GIVEN A DIAGNOSIS

Q: What exactly is wrong? What is my condition called?
A:

Q: If you recommend a **test** for further information, what do you expect to learn? (E.g. will an X-ray or
   MRI tell you about how severe the injury/tear/condition is?
A:

TREATMENT RECOMMENDATIONS

Q: What are your recommendations?   Short term?   Long term?
A:

If surgery is suggested:

Q: What are your main reasons for suggesting surgery? E.g. Increased range of motion?
   Decrease and/or eliminate pain now? Other?
A:

Q: What kind of surgery do you advise? What are the pros and cons of arthroscopic surgery and
   traditional surgery?
A:

QUESTIONS
for...

AN ORTHOPEDIST (cont'd.)

Q. When do you advise me to have surgery: Immediately?   Soon?   Later?
Please state your reasons.

A:

Q: How long might I expect to experience pain?

A:

Q: What kind of post-surgical pain management would I need? Pain pump?

A:

Q: How long after surgery can I start physical therapy?

A:

Q: How long will I need to curtail specific activities, such as walking, bending, lifting, driving, playing sports?

A:

Q: What can I expect to be able to do after my surgery…

A: In the first 6 weeks?_____

        1–3 months later? _____

        3–6 months later? _____

        And when can I resume my 'normal' life? _____

Q: What harm or danger is there if I don't have surgery?   Short-term?   Long-term?

A:

Q: How can I prevent my _____ muscles from deteriorating? If atrophy is possible, please
give me the time frame over which this would happen. What might I expect for each of the following?

        Short-term in a matter of months to a year? _____

        Mid-range 1–5 years ? _____

        Long-term—as part of the natural process of aging? _____

About physical therapy

Q: Is it possible that, with good physical therapy, surgery might be avoided in my case?

A:

Q: Can strengthening exercises help, such as those recommended by a chiropractor, sports coach or
physical therapist?   Do you recommend them?

A.

Q: What other treatment options might you suggest? For example, cold laser treatments?

A:

QUESTIONS
about...

KEEPING MY LIFESTYLE HEALTHY

Dr. _____ Date (mmddyyyy) _____

My specific health challenge _____

Identify the questions you would like to ask a health practitioner about healthy lifestyle habits to support your healing. Cross out those that do not apply. Add others as needed.

Nutrition:

Q: What foods are good for me and what should I avoid?   For example:

A: fruits   dairy   fish   soda

   vegetables   red meat   alcohol   gluten

   soy   poultry   tobacco   salt

   Foods that boost my immune system:

   Foods that help me stabilize my weight:

Exercise:

Q: What activities are safe for me to do, and what activities must I avoid?
A:

Q: How frequently and for how long should I exercise?
A:

Sleep:

Q: How many hours sleep do you recommend? Do you advise a catnap during the day when I'm not working?
A:

Weight:

Q: What is my ideal BMI (Body Mass Index)?
A:

Other support and resources:

Q: Would it be beneficial to work with a health practitioner who has been trained in a different perspective or modality?
A:

Q: Can you suggest any support groups / blogs / chat groups for my specific illness?
A:

Q: Please recommend a therapist, emotional counselor or spiritual guide who has experience with _____ patients OR other resources to support my emotional and spiritual wellbeing.
A:

Q: What can I do to reduce my stress and anxiety?
A:

QUESTIONS about...

MY PERSONAL WELLNESS COMMITMENTS

Date (mmddyyyy)_____

Review the healthy lifestyle suggestions you have received, and identify the commitments to good health you are now willing to make, by noting when you can you answer "yes" to any of the statements below.

1. I am eliminating as much stress as possible.

2. I have confidence in my doctors and in my treatment.

3. I will reach out to _____ for support.

4. I will persevere even when things are difficult.

5. I believe I will be among those who recover and heal from my illness.

6. I am now ready to make changes in my lifestyle to increase my chances of wellness, for example:

Check those that you can commit to at this time

- ☐ relaxation
- ☐ meditation
- ☐ guided imagery
- ☐ singing
- ☐ painting or being creative by _____
- ☐ listening to music
- ☐ appreciation of beauty
- ☐ connecting to nature
- ☐ walking
- ☐ exercise by _____
- ☐ wholesome diet, limiting / giving up alcohol, tobacco, sugar
- ☐ people I love to be with_____ _____
- ☐ things I love to do _____

- ☐ resurrecting an old hobby
- ☐ massage and / or body work
- ☐ having naps
- ☐ pampering myself by _____ _____
- ☐ writing in my journal*
- ☐ dreams—short-term and / or long-term goals _____
- ☐ laughter
- ☐ gratitude
- ☐ movies
- ☐ gardening
- ☐ time alone
- ☐ other ways to love and appreciate my life _____

Make a schedule with notes about how and *when* you will follow through on these choices.

A good time to review your wellness commitments is when you review your medical healthcare progress on p.62.

*This could also be a good time to re-read personal notes if you keep a journal. Some people find doing so really helpful.

Keep going step-by-step and congratulate yourself!

Remember to reach out to someone for encouragement and support when you need it.

QUESTIONS
for...

YOUR HEALTHCARE PRACTITIONER TOWARDS THE END OF TREATMENT

Dr. _____ Date (mmddyyyy) _____

Wellness After Treatment

Towards the end of treatment you may feel happy and relieved that your medical visits need not be as frequent. Yet you may be somewhat apprehensive without the monitoring and encouragement that regular visits to a trusted health professional have given you. It is beneficial to enlist your doctor's help to address any lingering health concerns you may have as you look towards the future. This will hopefully alleviate any sense you may have of being vulnerable, without an anchor, as you move forward.

Select the questions you would like to ask your doctor:

Future Professional Support

Q: Under what circumstances and how often should I come back to see you, my family doctor or _____ / another specialist or complementary practitioner?

A: **Who?**   **For what?**   **When?**

_____

_____

_____

Maintaining Good Health

Refer to _Keeping My Lifestyle Healthy_ (page 50) and _My Wellness Commitments_ (page 51) and list any questions you still wish to ask.

Q: Do you have any further suggestions regarding healthy lifestyle habits, given my health history?
A:

If you have any other concerns or need any further information, now is the time to speak up!

Q: Please address my concern: _____
A:

To Sum Up

Please prioritize your top three recommendations for your future health (or more if you wish):

1._____

2._____

3._____

QUESTIONS for...   MYSELF TOWARDS THE END OF TREATMENT

Personal Preferences and Support

Q: What are my top priorities, hopes, needs and intentions for my future health and well being?

1. _____

2. _____

3. _____

4. _____

5. _____

Balance your doctor's key suggestions with your own personal preferences and re-order your list above, if appropriate.

Q: Who would I like to ask to support me emotionally in order to put into practice the healthy lifestyle changes I am now choosing to make?

Name of Person	**Family/friend/health professional**	**Contact details**

Now decide to support your health as best you can!

Review your commitments regularly (monthly?) and renew, or change, to keep your plan as up-to-date as possible. Be sure to take it with you to any new appointments with your primary care doctor, gynecologist, and other specialists.

Don't forget to make your future life decisions.

Q: Have I taken care of all my future life choices (advance directives) to make my wishes clear about end of life health care and what I wish to pass on to others?

If not, immediately review pages 77 and 78 for guidance and take action to update your living will, health care proxy, will, and power of attorney. (This will ease your mind and be helpful to your family. Being prepared does not mean you are about to die.)

OTHER ADVANCE PREPARATION

❀ Mark all your appointments on a weekly or monthly calendar—paper or electronic, noting time, place, and practitioner. **Keep this calendar even *after* your appointments to verify your billing when it comes in.**

❀ Find out well ahead of time whether your doctor requires you to fill out any forms prior to your visit and whether he/ she has access to your electronic records. If not, provide any contact information necessary for a smooth transmission of vital information from another office and make sure to follow up as appropriate. Without your records, your doctor, or a medical specialist from another office, you may not be able to assess your situation properly.

❀ If your appointment is for a test, make sure you understand any pre-consultation instructions such as dietary restrictions.

A FEW PRETTY GOOD TIPS

FOR MY NEXT APPOINTMENT

Use the pocket inside the front cover of your binder as a temporary holding place where you can keep a folder for the papers you will need for an upcoming appointment.

Before each visit

❀ Ask yourself "What papers do I need to take with me?" These may include previous tests and reports you may need to refer to at your appointment.

❀ Select your reports, notes, questions for the practitioner, etc. Before you move them, pencil on them where they belong so that you can return them to the correct place.

❀ Place a sticky note as a page marker at the original location before moving any papers.

❀ Transfer your selected information to this pocket. For a second opinion consultation, it is likely that you will need most, or all, of your medical information. For follow-up visits with your regular doctor, you will need much less, especially if you have given him or her permission to make copies.

❀ Take your updated *My Yellow Pages* (especially your Emergency Contact Numbers and Chronological Health Log) to all your appointments.

After each visit

❀ Prepare the Medical Visit Worksheet on P. 57 and note the answers to your questions at the visit.

❀ Return the papers to their original location unless you need them for your next appointment.

ON APPOINTMENT DAYS

A FEW PRETTY GOOD TIPS

BEFORE YOU LEAVE HOME

Be sure to bring the papers you have gathered for your next appointment with you.

❀ Check if a support person is allowed to accompany you into the medical building. If so, plan accordingly and meet the family member, friend or local support group representative early enough to share your list of questions and talk together about the purpose of your visit, and the kind of support you would appreciate (if you have not already done so).

❀ Call the office beforehand to find out if the doctor is on schedule, or your appointment will be delayed due to an emergency. This is not unusual. You might be able to adjust your schedule.

❀ If you wish to record your visit, take a small recording device, ready for that possibility.

❀ Think about how best to take care of yourself while waiting. For example, choose a good book, magazine or bring along a portable music player with ear phones. You might also want a bottle of water and a shawl cover-up for the cold examining rooms.

Remember to bring your mask to wear indoors, if still mandated.

IN THE WAITING ROOM OR FRONT OFFICE

❀ On arrival, be friendly to the person at the front desk, and make a note of his or her name. A receptionist can be a helpful ally when you are making future appointments or when you have practical questions to ask. Introduce your companion. Confirm that you have permission for him/her to be present during the consultation.

❀ Relax with some deep breaths and feel your feet firmly on the ground.

❀ Ask the person accompanying you to be prepared to take notes for you and remind him or her of what you particularly wish the focus to be.

❀ Add any last minute questions to your list that arise while you are waiting.

❀ If something is bothering you, such as a noisy TV or insufficient ventilation, and you are really uncomfortable, ask the office receptionist if there's a way to remedy the situation.

❀ Check if the doctor is going to be delayed. If so, consider a walk or wait in your car, the hospital cafeteria or a local cafe. Check back just before the anticipated adjusted time or, before you leave the waiting room, request that the receptionist call your cell phone when the health professional is almost ready to see you.

A FEW PRETTY GOOD TIPS

IN THE CONSULTING ROOM— OR DURING A TELEMEDICINE VISIT.*

INITIAL CONNECTIONS AND QUESTIONS

Any reference to a companion assumes that you will follow current guidelines.

❀ If your anxiety level is high, when entering the office, remind yourself that that you have prepared well, have your list of questions with you and the person accompanying you is there to support you. Even if you don't always hear or remember everything that is being said, your companion will catch things you might miss. Ask your companion to write the answers to your questions so you can keep breathing—and stay present.

❀ Ask the physician for permission to record the consultation, especially if a support person is not allowed to be with you..

❀ Listen to what the doctor has to say. Note any questions that arise while you are listening and ask your companion to check off those that have been addressed. Ask for clarification whenever you feel you need it.

❀ Go through your list of questions and ask all of them systematically.

❀ If you feel rushed, breathe deeply again and ask the health practitioner to slow down. Ask your companion if she/he understands the gist of what is being said, and to rephrase the answer back to you to make sure you understand it.

❀ Feeling that you are interviewing your doctor may also boost your confidence. Your questions are NOT an imposition on your health providers. Questions help practitioners to know more about you, so that they can do a better job.

❀ If your physician doesn't appear to be listening to you or is not willing to answer your questions, that person may not be the best professional for you.

❀ **Do *not* sign up for treatment on the spot. You need time to integrate what you have heard before you come to a decision.**

*TELEMEDICINE enables the remote diagnosis, treatment and follow-up of patients by means of telecommunications technology, using HIPPA compliant video-conferencing tools.

MEDICAL VISIT WORKSHEET

Some medical offices provide a printout of a "Clinical Visit Summary of Today's Visit". If not, use this form.

Visit to _____ Reason for visit _____

Initial routine check-in with _____

Vital signs: Weight _____ Temperature: _____ Blood pressure _____

Pulse: _____ Blood count _____ Other _____

Meeting with _____ MD

Nurse Practitioner/ Specialist / Other _____

My update (since last diagnosis) _____

_____

Comments in response _____

_____

My concerns _____

_____

Comments in response _____

_____

My questions _____

_____

_____

_____

Answers given _____

_____

_____

Follow up suggestions / next steps _____

_____

_____

_____

_____

NOTES

PART 4

FOLLOWING UP AFTER APPOINTMENTS

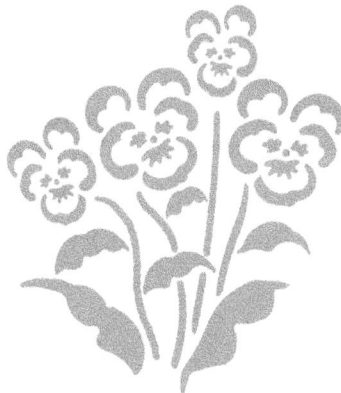

AFTER MY MEDICAL APPOINTMENTS
Organize your notes while your memory is still fresh.

SUMMARIZE YOUR PRIORITIES **on the next page after every health care visit whether at a conventional or complementary practitioner's office or at a hospital.**

❊ Identify each meeting clearly with the medical professional's name and the date.

❊ Note any matters that you want to follow-up—further research, reading, or interviews. Include your personal observations and impressions. Add self-care (non-medical) ideas that you might also wish to explore.

❊ Update any decisions.

Update your medical history in your *Chronological Health History* after every visit. It will become a useful reference for all your practitioners, as well as for yourself.

Make a note of your next appointment in your calendar.

Complete your *Review and Update Medical Healthcare Progress* (pages 62–63) on a regular basis. As you review your progress, renew your commitment to good health. Remind yourself that your health is in your hands as well as your doctor's. You can use your mind, emotions, and spirit to help your body heal.

A FEW PRETTY GOOD TIPS

GETTING THE ANSWERS YOU NEED

❊ **Review with your companion your Q. and A. notes of what was said and the course of action suggested by the professional, *as soon after your appointment as possible.*** Details can fade very fast, especially if you did not record the appointment. Underline the important points the doctor made about your diagnosis, his or her answers, and recommendations. If you are not sure about any aspect of the discussion or if your perceptions differ greatly from those of the person accompanying you, identify the area of confusion and reframe a question to clarify it.

❊ Consider sending these subsequent questions to your doctor's office for attention. If your writing is very difficult to read, type or ask someone to type key information / questions.

❊ If you come away from an appointment sensing your questions were not being addressed, or you are not clear about an explanation, don't consider your lack of understanding as unintelligent or your doubts as silly. Honor them as contributing to your well-being—and note questions you now wish to ask. If necessary, talk to someone from a support group or online chatroom who understands medical implications / terminology.

SUMMARIZE PRIORITIES AFTER EVERY HEALTHCARE VISIT

Dr. _____Date (mmddyyyy) _____

Preferred way to be contacted: _____

MY DOCTOR'S, OR OTHER PROFESSIONAL'S, MOST IMPORTANT RECOMMENDATIONS

To do now:

"Down the line" recommendations for later:

MY RESPONSE

After reviewing my experience and my notes, THE MOST IMPORTANT OUTCOMES of this

appointment are: _____

_____

My predominant feelings are: _____

_____

Follow-up actions I might take:

> Schedule an additional test? YES / NO
>
> Get a second opinion / see another practitioner?   YES / NO
>
> Schedule a recommended treatment?   For what?_____When? _____
>
> Explore further research?   YES / NO
>
> Check out other resources recommended?   YES / NO
>
> Postpone any follow-up until I have further information or additional test results? YES / NO
>
> Do I need more information about technical / medical words, procedures, etc. that I don't fully understand?   YES / NO

IF YES to any questions, note when and how to follow up…

My impressions of the practitioner, staff and the facility:

> Strengths? E.g. welcoming, friendly, professional, knowledgeable? _____
>
> Practitioner's capacity to listen and communicate answers to my questions clearly? _____
>
> Other? _____
>
> Weaknesses? E.g. preoccupied or impatient staff; stuffy or noisy facility? _____
>
> Other? _____

❧ **Do I wish to continue with this professional?   YES / NO**

REVIEW AND UPDATE MEDICAL HEALTHCARE PROGRESS

Weekly, monthly or whenever you wish to take an inventory of your progress.

Reviewing your medical healthcare progress after a number of visits will give you an overview of a bigger picture and you will notice if anything is falling through the cracks.

FOR THE PERIOD FROM _____ TO _____

What are the most significant ideas to have emerged from consultations / conversations?

How might I follow-up these ideas?

PROGRESS

Is there an overall treatment plan in place?

- If not, who can help me put one in place?

- If so, how is this plan progressing?

- What specific progress has been made since my last review?

Is my treatment plan proceeding in a timely manner?

- Do I feel rushed to make decisions?

- Am I satisfied with the rate of progress?

REVIEW AND UPDATE MEDICAL HEALTHCARE PROGRESS (Cont'd)

COMMUNICATION

✌ Am I being kept informed? Am I sufficiently included in the decision-making loop?

• Have reports been sent to the practitioners I have so requested?

• Are my health care providers communicating about, and coordinating, my treatment?

• If not, where specifically is coordination lacking?

CURRENT TREATMENT GOALS FROM _____ UNTIL _____

✌ What are my treatment goals?

• For next week? Beginning date   _____

• Next month? Beginning date   _____

• Three months hence? From_____ to _____

OTHER OBSERVATIONS

✌ How do I feel?

• How is my body responding to treatment?

• Am I experiencing any fatigue, aches, pains, unusual body sensations or any differences in my sleep pattern?

Check often that your treatment log is fully up-to-date and that you have noted all upcoming appointments in your calendar.

When you review your medical health care progress, take a moment to review your personal wellness commitments also.

ORGANIZE DOCTORS' PAPERWORK

Identify all your currently active doctors and health care practitioners.

Your active team might include your primary care physician, surgeon, gynecologist, healer, oncologist, nutritionist, cardiologist, chiropractor, urologist, endocrinologist, auto-immune specialist, acupuncturist, naturopath, or massage therapist.

Organize each practitioner's papers separately.

Arrange each set of papers in dated order, with the most recent report on top.

Remember to add the date mm/dd/**yyyy**. (Especially the year).

For each, include records of all consultations or visits, your preparatory questions, doctors' answers, your follow-up notes, and prescriptions or recommendations you receive.

Create a tab divider for each practitioner and arrange them in alphabetical order or whatever way works for you.

A FEW PRETTY GOOD TIPS

SO MANY DOCTORS, SO MANY TABS

You may be surprised at the number of specialists you may be asked to consult, and in addition, you may have complementary care appointments. You don't need to use a separate tab for everyone in an office. (i.e. All paperwork with regard to your primary care physician, his or her nurse, physician's assistant, and receptionist would go in your primary care physician's section.)

If you are interested in, or are combining, both conventional medicine and complementary care, divide your information into two parts: one for conventional and another for complementary. If you are seeing an integrative doctor, keep both parts together.

If you have enrolled in any Online Patient Portals, keep a clear record of its name and the information you can access, along with your password for each.

Note: Do not include financial or legal papers along with your medical papers. It is more efficient to keep them separately; perhaps in another secure place.

ORGANIZE TESTS, REPORTS AND MEDICATIONS

Identify tests you have had such as blood work, x-rays, scans, pathology and consultation records; and ask your doctor or hospital to provide copies of results once they are available.

Fill out the pages for:

Results from laboratories and other facilities

Medications, pharmacies and other suppliers

Vitamins, minerals, supplements and suppliers

Put medical reports and test results from each type of test together with your notes, in dated order, most recent on top, and file them behind the appropriate divider.

For example, keep radiology and blood work reports separate from each other within this section. It will then be easier to reference them at your next visit or set of tests.

FILING YOUR REPORTS

In the beginning it may not seem necessary to separate the reports, but later it becomes essential as more and more information will come your way.

- ❀ Highlight the date of test results or lab-work mm/dd/**yyyy** (Remember the year).

- ❀ Add notes you have made related to going for tests and receiving results.

Keep medical release forms and privacy statements connected to these tests with your legal records.

*The use of "certified" **Electronic Health Records (EHRs)** is almost universally in place in hospitals and physicians' offices, so that patient records can be easily transmitted as needed. Since 2016 all health care providers are required to make electronic copies of patient records available to patients, at their request, in machine-readable form. (The 21st Century Cures Act.).

In this digital age, it is highly unlikely that you will be asked to transport your records from one doctor to another for an upcoming appt.

RESULTS FROM LABORATORIES AND OTHER FACILITIES GIVING REPORTS

Name of lab or facility _____ | TEST _____

Contact person _____ | Date (mmddyyyy) _____

Address _____ | Reason _____

Tel _____ Fax _____ Email _____ | Results _____

Best way to contact _____ | Filed? Yes / No

Name of lab or facility _____ | TEST _____

Contact person _____ | Date _____

Address _____ | Reason _____

Tel _____ Fax _____ Email _____ | Results _____

Best way to contact _____ | Filed? Yes / No

Name of lab or facility _____ | TEST _____

Contact person _____ | Date _____

Address _____ | Reason _____

Tel _____ Fax _____ Email _____ | Results _____

Best way to contact _____ | Filed? Yes / No

Name of lab or facility _____ | TEST _____

Contact person _____ | Date _____

Address _____ | Reason _____

Tel _____ Fax _____ Email _____ | Results _____

Best way to contact _____ | Filed? Yes / No

Name of lab or facility _____ | TEST _____

Contact person _____ | Date _____

Address _____ | Reason _____

Tel _____ Fax _____ Email _____ | Results _____

Best way to contact _____ | Filed? Yes / No

Name of lab or facility _____ | TEST _____

Contact person _____ | Date _____

Address _____ | Reason _____

Tel _____ Fax _____ Email _____ | Results _____

Best way to contact _____ | Filed? Yes / No

MEDICATION AND PHARMACIES / SUPPLIERS

For each medication note the following information:

Name of medication _____ Circle: generic / brand | **Pharmacy or supplier:**

Prescribed by_____ Date **(mmddyyyy)**_____ | _____

For_____Dosage _____ | Contact person _____

Date began _____Instructions _____ | Address _____

Doctors informed of new prescription _____ | Best way to contact: _____

Positive/negative results/side effects _____ | _____

Name of medication _____ Circle: generic / brand | **Pharmacy or supplier:**

Prescribed by_____ Date _____ | _____

For_____Dosage _____ | Contact person _____

Date began _____Instructions _____ | Address _____

Doctors informed of new prescription _____ | Best way to contact: _____

Positive/negative results/side effects _____ | _____

Name of medication _____ Circle: generic / brand | **Pharmacy or supplier:**

Prescribed by_____ Date _____ | _____

For_____Dosage _____ | Contact person _____

Date began _____Instructions _____ | Address _____

Doctors informed of new prescription _____ | Best way to contact: _____

Positive/negative results/side effects _____ | _____

Name of medication _____ Circle: generic / brand | **Pharmacy or supplier:**

Prescribed by_____ Date _____ | _____

For_____Dosage _____ | Contact person _____

Date began _____Instructions _____ | Address _____

Doctors informed of new prescription _____ | Best way to contact: _____

Positive/negative results/side effects _____ | _____

Name of medication _____ Circle: generic / brand | **Pharmacy or supplier:**

Prescribed by_____ Date _____ | _____

For_____Dosage _____ | Contact person _____

Date began _____Instructions _____ | Address _____

Doctors informed of new prescription _____ | Best way to contact: _____

Positive/negative results/side effects _____ | _____

VITAMINS, MINERALS, SUPPLEMENTS AND SUPPLIERS

For each vitamin, mineral or supplement, note the following information:

Name of vitamin/supplement _____ | **Manufacturer** _____

Authorized by _____ Date (mmddyyyy) _____ | **Source of supply:**

For_____Dosage _____ | Health Food Store_____

Date began _____Instructions _____ | Pharmacy _____

Doctors/practitioners informed of supplement _____ | Online _____

Positive/negative results/side effects _____ | _____

Name of vitamin/supplement _____ | **Manufacturer** _____

Authorized by _____ Date _____ | **Source of supply:**

For_____Dosage _____ | Health Food Store_____

Date began _____Instructions _____ | Pharmacy _____

Doctors/practitioners informed of supplement _____ | Online _____

Positive/negative results/side effects _____ | _____

Name of vitamin/supplement _____ | **Manufacturer** _____

Authorized by _____ Date _____ | **Source of supply:**

For_____Dosage _____ | Health Food Store_____

Date began _____Instructions _____ | Pharmacy _____

Doctors/practitioners informed of supplement _____ | Online _____

Positive/negative results/side effects _____ | _____

Name of vitamin/supplement _____ | **Manufacturer** _____

Authorized by _____ Date _____ | **Source of supply:**

For_____Dosage _____ | Health Food Store_____

Date began _____Instructions _____ | Pharmacy _____

Doctors/practitioners informed of supplement _____ | Online _____

Positive/negative results/side effects _____ | _____

Name of vitamin/supplement _____ | **Manufacturer** _____

Authorized by _____ Date _____ | **Source of supply:**

For_____Dosage _____ | Health Food Store_____

Date began _____Instructions _____ | Pharmacy _____

Doctors/practitioners informed of supplement _____ | Online _____

Positive/negative results/side effects _____ | _____

PART 5

BILLS, INSURANCE AND LEGAL RECORDS

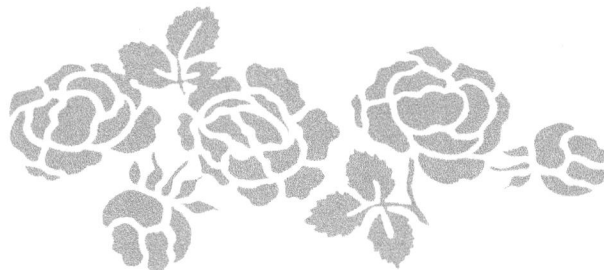

ORGANIZE BILLS

It is highly unlikely that you will need to bring any papers pertaining to billing to your medical appointments. Consider keeping all your financial papers, including bills in clearly marked folders in a drawer of a filing cabinet or in a firebox. Keep them separate from other medical notes pertaining to health practitioners or test results. If you do wish to keep them in a separate binder, use divider tabs and clear sheet protectors or pockets.

MAKE AND RECORD PAYMENTS

First, separate out UNPAID bills and PAID bills.

UNPAID BILLS (PENDING):

Put all your unpaid bills in the *UNPAID BILLS* section until they have been paid and acknowledged as paid. Review regularly.

Place an urgent bill in a special section or folder earmarked for that purpose with a name such as "IMMEDIATE ATTENTION," and keep it in an obvious place where you cannot forget it. Then take action as soon as you can.

Keep doctors' bills together with insurance bills if you have health insurance, since health providers and insurance companies are closely connected through billing practices.

And especially separate out UNPAID BILLS from PAID BILLS if you and your insurance are each paying a portion.

PAID BILLS:

Use the *PAID BILLS* section when NO further payment is required in connection with the charge. As your bills are completed and accumulate, consider transferring them to a separate folder/ binder marked "Completed" as you don't need to take them to appointments.

DIVIDE YOUR PAID BILLS into the following 3 categories behind the appropriate dividers:

1. Non-reimbursable Bills—You alone are responsible for paying these bills.

2. Reimbursable Bills (Primary Insurance) You expect your primary insurance company to pay in part or in whole.

File here only those primary insurance bills that require *no* further payment in connection with the charge.

Put these bills together in dated order, most recent on top.

3. Reimbursable Bills (Secondary Insurance) You expect your secondary insurance company to pay in part or in whole.

File your secondary insurance bills when it is clear that *no* further payment is required in connection with the charge.

Put these bills together in dated order, most recent on top.

PAYING BILLS

* **Check thoroughly before you pay any bill.** Sometimes statements are very confusing and often arrive quite a long time after your actual appointment. Some charges are even incorrect. Refer to your medical calendar to check that the date on the bill corresponds to the date of the appointment.

* **Make a copy of the bill and file it before paying.** Note on the bill the date on which you paid it, the check number, and the name of any person you spoke to in connection with the payment.

* **Ask for help if you are not confident about interpreting bills**—contact the person in the billing department of your physician's office, or a social worker.

* **Keep accurate copies of all medical bills, insurance statements (often called Explanation of Benefits or EOB's) and receipts.** This will serve you well when it's tax time.

TAX DEDUCTIONS

❀ Ask a tax preparer or financial adviser about tax deductions in connection with your illness and the information they will need from you.

❀ Keep a monthly tally of all your expenses as follows. (It will be easier at the end of the year):

Monthly

Premium payments	$ _____
Travel expenses	$ _____
Co-pay	$ _____
Co-insurance	$ _____
Prescriptions	$ _____
Total	$ _____

Annual

Total premium payments	$ _____
Total travel expenses	$ _____
Total co-pay	$ _____
Total co-insurance	$ _____
Total prescriptions	$ _____
Annual insurance deductible	$ _____
Total	$ _____

❀ Subtract any payments reimbursed by your insurance company, as you will not be able to claim them.

❀ Keep an accurate record of all your medical expenses for the IRS in order to claim them on your tax return. Note mileage and keep all gas, toll, hotel, meal, rail, bus and airline receipts for every health related journey, as well as other out-of-pocket expenses such as prescription drugs and medical equipment.

A FEW PRETTY GOOD TIPS

ORGANIZE INSURANCE CLAIMS AND RECORDS

USE THE *WHAT MY INSURANCE COVERS* FORM (page 74) to clarify exactly what you can expect from your Insurance Companies or include a copy of your policies in your binder.

FILL OUT *MY CONTACTS WITH INSURANCE COMPANIES* FORM (page 75) to record all contacts with your insurance company, including calls, emails and letters. Attach copies of any correspondence or forms submitted.

Enter your insurance information, including membership I.D., plan name and policy numbers for all your insurance carriers, in your Yellow Pages.

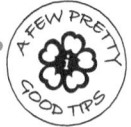

KNOW YOUR POLICY

Review your policy/policies carefully, *before* you get any treatment. Annual deductibles, co-payments per office visit, test, prescription drugs (brand name and generic), ambulance service, or wellness care allowed can vary greatly.

Many different types of health plans exist, including group plans, individual plans, HMO's, disability income insurance, long-term care plans, Medicaid, and for seniors—Medicare. An HMO policy requires you to choose a local participating doctor or facility, or pay out of pocket non-reimbursable expenses for services outside your network plan.

The right kind of coverage should provide benefits for in-patient hospital care, physician services, lab work and X-rays, prescription drugs, outpatient services and nursing home care at a location of your choice. If necessary, get help from your insurance provider to understand your plan.

A FEW PRETTY GOOD TIPS

WHAT MY INSURANCE COVERS (PRIMARY AND SUPPLEMENTARY)

My outpatient benefits are:

My inpatient benefits are:

What are the different co-payments or percentage co-insurance I have to make for

Inpatient?_____   Specialist? _____

Outpatient? _____   Mental health practitioner?_____

Primary care physician?_____   My annual deductible? _____

What % do I have to pay after my annual deductible is met?_____

What is the maximum life-time benefit / cap, if any? _____

How do I file a claim?

Do I have out-of-network benefits? If so, what is the co-pay? _____

Will my insurance cover the following?

Second opinions?   YES / NO   Home healthcare?   YES / NO

Clinical trials?   YES / NO   Other _____ ?   YES / NO

If yes, do I need a referral, and from whom? _____

When must I get preauthorization for treatment or consultations? _____

If pre-authorization is required, who has to make the treatment referral? _____

MY CONTACTS WITH INSURANCE COMPANIES

To/From: _____(Person contacted) **Insurance company** _____

Tel. #_____ Ext._____

Date(mmddyyyy) _____ Time_____ **Claim/reference number** _____

Question, issue or dispute discussed _____

_____

Answer/action needed/ agreed _____

_____

To/From: _____(Person contacted) **Insurance company** _____

Tel. #_____ Ext._____

Date(mmddyyyy) _____ Time_____ **Claim/reference number** _____

Question, issue or dispute discussed _____

_____

Answer/action needed/ agreed _____

_____

To/From: _____(Person contacted) **Insurance company** _____

Tel. #_____ Ext._____

Date(mmddyyyy) _____ Time_____ **Claim/reference number** _____

Question, issue or dispute discussed _____

_____

Answer/action needed/ agreed _____

_____

To/From: _____(Person contacted) **Insurance company** _____

Tel. #_____ Ext._____

Date(mmddyyyy) _____ Time_____ **Claim/reference number** _____

Question, issue or dispute discussed _____

_____

Answer/action needed/ agreed _____

_____

SUBMITTING CLAIMS

At your first visit, expect health care providers to ask for and make a copy of your current insurance card(s) and your driver's license or State approved ID. Ask whether they will submit a claim on your behalf or whether you will have to do this yourself. If they agree to submit your claim, and you don't receive paperwork in a timely fashion, say three weeks, check in with them to make sure they have followed through.

If necessary, get help filing claims. Some insurance companies have case managers. In a situation where you are likely to have on-going contact with your insurer, ask if they will assign a case manager to you. That's not always possible, so if you find yourself talking to a particularly helpful representative, thank that person, **request his or her name and telephone extension,** and ask to be connected to that extension in future calls.

If you don't understand a bill or an Explanation of Benefits or if the amount is different from what you expect, keep asking questions. **Insurance companies can make mistakes. Be persistent.**

If your insurance company rejects a claim that has been submitted, call the company to ask their representative why it was rejected. Then immediately call the billing person in your medical professional's office. Explain what the insurance representative told you and ask them to look into the matter on your behalf. If you are still not satisfied, don't give up—file again. A wrong code for your diagnosis is a common error. Other reasons a claim is denied include a decision that your procedure was not medically necessary, that you have a pre-existing condition, that it is a "non-covered" benefit or that you have chosen to go "out-of-network."

If a claim you still understand to be justified is again rejected, request the insurance company's appeal process and make an appeal. Ask someone to review your letter before you send it in to make sure it is clear and accurate.

If you feel that the insurance company is inappropriately handling your case, or if you have a continuing unresolved dispute, lodge a complaint with your state's Insurance Department. You may be able to do this online. For example, New York State residents can go to www.ins.state.ny.us. A local Legal Aid office might also help.

Don't get discouraged.
Take a break, go for a walk, have a cup of tea, call up a friend, ask for help and come back to it later.

ORGANIZE LEGAL PAPERS

Divide your legal records behind the dividers for CURRENT TREATMENT and FUTURE LIFE CHOICES.

❋ **CURRENT TREATMENT:** You will be asked to sign many different types of forms.

> **Sub-divide the following as you receive them:**
>> ❋ Consent forms for treatment
>>
>> ❋ Medical release forms
>>
>> ❋ Privacy statements
>>
>> ❋ Other legal papers

> **DO NOT SIGN ANY CONSENT FORMS, if the exact procedure has not been described or if you do not understand it. Your consent must be fully informed.**

> Cross out statements that are not in agreement with your wishes. Even if your doctor has forceful opinions and strong recommendations, it is your decision and responsibility, as a mentally competent adult, to accept or refuse treatment.

> Consider keeping consent forms and medical release forms in a separate binder as you will rarely refer to them.

> Consider keeping important papers in a fire-proof box.

❋ **FUTURE LIFE CHOICES: Advance directives** ensure your wishes are as binding as possible concerning end-of-life issues and what you wish to pass onto your loved ones. (See page 78 for details of legal and non-binding advance directives.)

> **Make sure you fill out the following legal forms AS SOON AS POSSIBLE**, if you have not already done so. This will make it easy for yourself and your loved ones at a later date:
>> ❋ Living Will*
>>
>> ❋ Health Care Proxy* or Agent (health care power of attorney)
>>
>> ❋ Will
>>
>> ❋Power of Attorney

> **Search the Internet to download state-specific forms that will be honored as legal if properly signed.**

> Note who has a copy of each in *My Yellow Pages*, once you have filled them out.

---

* When preparing your Living Will and your Healthcare Proxy, I highly recommend "FIVE WISHES," available from www.agingwithdignity.org 1-888-5-WISHES / 1-888-594-7437. The Five Wishes are for: "1. The person I want to make care decisions for me when I can't; 2. The kind of medical treatment I want or don't want; 3. How comfortable I want to be; 4. How I want people to treat me; and 5. What I want my loved ones to know."

LEGAL ADVANCE DIRECTIVES

These include

Health care proxy—delegating authority to another person to make health care decisions on your behalf, if you become mentally or physically incapacitated.

Living will—expressing your wishes, to guide your healthcare proxy, as to what your medical treatment should be. For example, you might wish to receive all possible medical interventions or you might refuse treatment that will artificially prolong your life. As previously stated, it's your right to decide to request or refuse treatment as a mentally competent adult.

Granting power of attorney—for non-health issues such as financial and other personal matters.

Writing a will or creating a trust—transferring your assets in accordance with your desires as opposed to your assets being transferred pursuant to state law.

It is wise to consult an attorney to ensure that any documents you have downloaded from the Internet **are in accordance with your state laws** and court precedents (not federal law).

❀ Give a copy of your living will to all significant family members, your doctors, your healthcare proxy and your lawyer. Make sure *everyone* knows about your decision to accept or decline treatment that will artificially prolong your life. It simply isn't enough to sign a living will and have it filed away.

❀ List where you keep these important documents in *My Yellow Pages*, Page 13.

Preparing advance directives does not mean you are about to die. Life will be much easier for your beloved family members and friends if they know your wishes.

NON-BINDING ADVANCE DIRECTIVES

Prepare non-binding advance directives at your leisure such as:

❀ Ethical Will (heartfelt thoughts, passing on your love and beliefs to family members and friends)

❀ Other papers (letters or gifts to specific individuals)

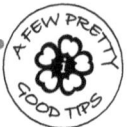

PART 6

MY REFERENCE LIBRARY

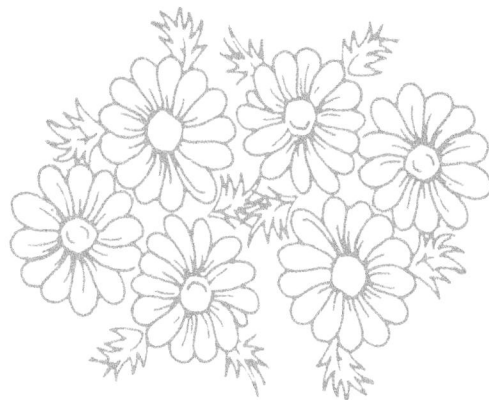

RESOURCES AND INFORMATION

Start to collect resources *at your own pace.*

Your resources might include information about:
- Organizations (health / community etc), internet and websites, newsletters and magazines
- Books, audios and videos, consulting, treatment information and referral services
- Research reports and articles, internet search engines, sources and information
- Sources of less expensive vitamins, organic produce, drugs
- Humor: movies, cartoons
- Personal anecdotes and miscellaneous resources

Use the organizing pages and tabs to divide information as best suits you.
- People and organizations to contact
- Good ideas from conversations / emails
- Suggestions to remember
- Favorite resources

A FEW PRETTY GOOD TIPS

There is a lot of information out there in all shapes and sizes, especially on the internet. It can be overpowering and possibly incorrect. If you are a person who is reassured by having a lot of information, you will be comfortable gathering it. Helpful guidelines for evaluating websites can be found at   http://medlineplus.gov/healthywebsurfing.html

Initially, you'll be able to put the material at the back of your organizer. Quite soon, you may find it necessary to sort it according to topic and place it in folders, file boxes or filing cabinet drawers.

If you are easily overwhelmed by lots of facts and figures, delegate this task to someone else.

PEOPLE AND ORGANIZATIONS TO CONTACT

List each person or organization you've heard about, and might like to contact at some point.

Name_____

Organization _____

Address (if known) _____

Tel/email/web site (if known) _____

Reason for contacting_____

Where I found out about this_____

Name_____

Organization _____

Address (if known) _____

Tel/email/web site (if known) _____

Reason for contacting_____

Where I found out about this_____

Name_____

Organization _____

Address (if known) _____

Tel/email/web site (if known) _____

Reason for contacting_____

Where I found out about this_____

Name_____

Organization _____

Address (if known) _____

Tel/email/web site (if known) _____

Reason for contacting_____

Where I found out about this_____

Name_____

Organization _____

Address (if known) _____

Tel/email/web site (if known) _____

Reason for contacting_____

Where I found out about this_____

GOOD IDEAS FROM CONVERSATIONS AND EMAILS

If you receive a helpful email, print it out and insert it with your resources / information.

Contact with (name of person) _____ On (date)_____

We discussed _____

New ideas / significant information_____

_____

I'll follow-up by _____

Contact with (name of person) _____ On (date)_____

We discussed _____

New ideas / significant information_____

_____

I'll follow-up by _____

Contact with (name of person) _____ On (date)_____

We discussed _____

New ideas / significant information_____

_____

I'll follow-up by _____

Contact with (name of person) _____ On (date)_____

We discussed _____

New ideas / significant information_____

_____

I'll follow-up by _____

Contact with (name of person) _____ On (date)_____

We discussed _____

New ideas / significant information_____

_____

I'll follow-up by _____

FAVORITE RESOURCES

If you use a computer for record keeping, note where this information is stored.

Articles

Books / Ebooks

Magazines

FAVORITE RESOURCES (cont'd)

Web sites

Advocacy organizations

National organizations

Other—such as medical research organizations

Local or hospital libraries

Blogs

AFTERWORD

My wish is that My Health & Wellness Organizer eases your process and lightens your load as you meet the various challenges following an initial diagnosis, a recurrence, or as you help a loved one with his/her medical journey and paperwork.

Blessings,
Puja Thomson

Thank you for purchasing
My Health & Wellness Organizer

2022 Revised Edition
ISBN 978-1-928663-14-0 $19.95

My Health & Wellness Organizer is also available from Roots & Wings as an
E-book in downloadable PDF format $7.95

Other titles from ROOTS & WINGS:

Track Your Truth—Discover Your Authentic Self
Paperback ISBN 978-1-928663-10-2 $17.95   E-book ISBN 978-1-928663-16-4 $4.95

After Shock: From Cancer Diagnosis to Healing (Second revised edition 2021)
Paperback ISBN 978-1-928663-17-1 $19.95

Roots & Wings for Strength and Freedom
Guided imagery and meditations to transform your life

- CD   ISBN 978-1-928663-08-9 $15.00
- MP3 (check online at rootsnwings.com/store)
- Paperback workbook Revised Edition   ISBN 978-1-928663-06-5 $19.95
- Workbook & CD Revised Edition   ISBN 978-1-928663-07-2 $24.00

My Hope & Focus Cancer Organizer
Second Revised edition 2022   ISBN 978-1-928663-15-7 $19.95
Also available as an e-book in downloadable PDF format from Roots & Wings for $7.95

TO ORDER
Any of the above titles or for general inquiries:

845-255-2278
www.rootsnwings.com/store
Also available from local bookstores and online retailers.

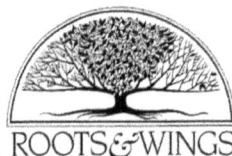

ROOTS & WINGS PUBLISHING
P. O. Box 1081, New Paltz, NY 12561   info@rootsnwings.com